Natural antibiotic and antiviral herbs

Making Use of Herbal Remedies to Fight Infections

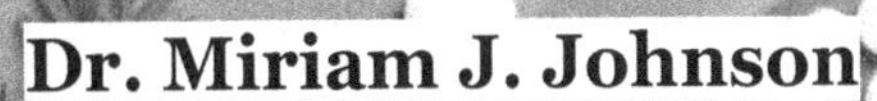

Abstract

Are you looking for natural alternatives to efficiently battle infections? Are you tired of the limits and potential hazards connected with standard antibiotics and antivirals?

If you're ready to take responsibility for your health and learn about the healing power of natural herbs, "Natural Antibiotic and Antiviral Herbs" is the book for you.

In this lengthy overview, we will examine three main obstacles that people encounter when trying to control infections:

Limited efficacy: Conventional therapy may not always give the expected effects. Are you looking for new techniques to boost your capacity to cure illnesses effectively?

Drug resistance: The emergence of drug-resistant bacteria and viruses is a serious concern. Do you worry about antibiotics and antivirals being less effective? Do you want to look at methods that can help lower the chance of resistance development?

Negative consequences: Conventional drugs frequently have unwanted side effects. Are you looking for safer alternatives that can help you prevent bad responses and improve your general well-being?

Here are five compelling reasons why "Natural Antibiotics and Antiviral Herbs" are the greatest solution to these issues:

In-depth knowledge: Learn about the mechanisms of action and the qualities of natural herbs. Learn how they can treat diseases and strengthen your body's defense mechanisms.

Discover practical and successful methods for incorporating natural herbs into your daily life. This book includes a range of ways to introduce these herbs into daily routine, including herbal combinations, meal planning, and recipes for breakfast, lunch, dinner, desserts, and snacks.

Expert advice: Take use of the skills of well-known specialists in the industry. This book is supported by the most recent research and scientific data, ensuring that you receive accurate and dependable information.

Consider taking a comprehensive strategy for infection therapy. Investigate the synergistic advantages of herbal combinations, increase the performance of your immune system, and manage your body's inflammatory response.

Personalized solutions: Recognize the relevance of individual variances and comprehend how genetic variables, health concerns, and concurrent drugs may influence your reaction to herbal medicines.

When you glance at the table of contents, you'll discover that some interesting chapters are waiting for you. Expect to learn about the benefits and limitations of natural herbs, as well as their mechanisms of action and how they could assist your body battle diseases.

You can expect a thorough guide on incorporating natural herbs into your daily routine with the accompanying breakfast, lunch, dinner, dessert, and snack recipes, as well as a 30-Day diet plan. Consider having tasty and gratifying meals while harnessing the power of these herbs to improve your health and well-being.

It's time to take action and boost your infection-control approach. Buy "Natural Antibiotic and Antiviral Herbs" immediately and start living a better, more natural lifestyle.

Don't put it off any longer. Your health deserves the highest possible treatment. Order your book today and learn the healing power of natural herbs.

Table Of Content

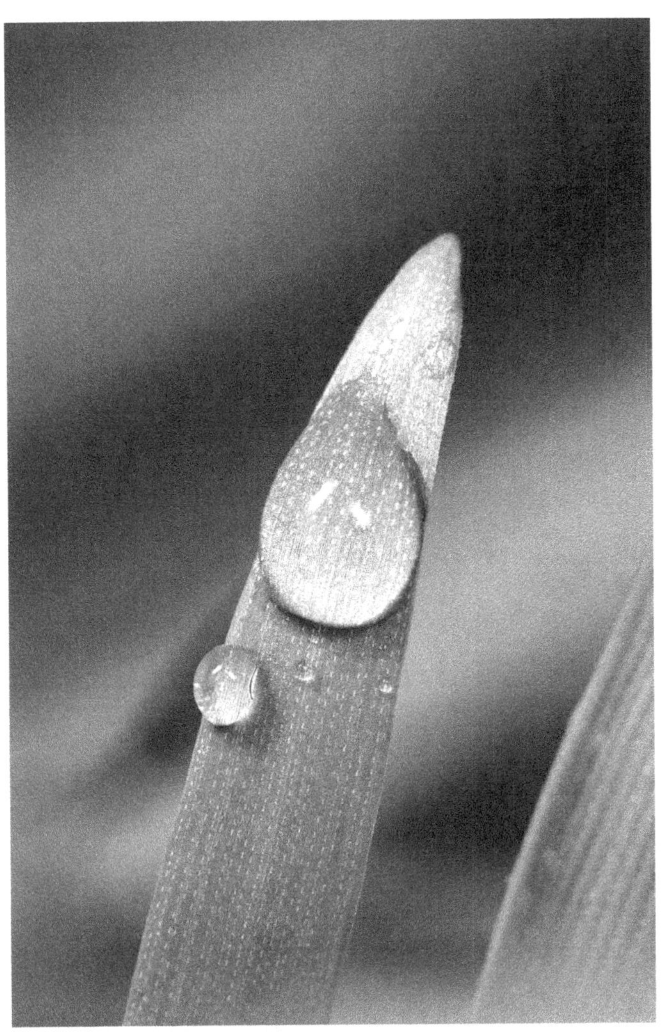

Introduction

Antibiotics and Antivirals: What Are Their Roles?

When hazardous bacteria or viruses penetrate our bodies, antibiotics, and antivirals help us fight them off. Let us analyze their purpose and functions:

Antibiotics: These drugs are meant to treat bacterial infections. Bacteria can cause a range of ailments, including urinary tract infections, strep throat, and pneumonia. Antibiotics operate by targeting and destroying bacteria or slowing their growth, allowing our immune system to more effectively tackle the infection.

Antivirals, as opposed to antibiotics, are used to treat viral illnesses. Viruses, such as the flu or common cold viruses, invade our cells and grow, producing sickness.

Antivirals suppress viral replication, which lessens the severity and duration of viral infections. They aid in the decrease of symptoms, the speeding up of healing, and the prevention of difficulties.

Antibiotics and antivirals are both crucial instruments in the medical armory against infections, but they have different purposes. Antibiotics cure bacterial infections, whereas antivirals treat viral ones. To enhance effectiveness, it is vital to utilize the appropriate type of medication for each unique infection.

It is crucial to understand, however, that antibiotics and antivirals only operate against bacteria and viruses, respectively. They are useless against other illnesses, such as fungal or parasitic infections. Different sorts of drugs or therapy may be required in distinct instances.

Remember that antibiotics and antivirals are recommended by healthcare professionals, and it is vital to strictly follow their directions. Misuse or overuse of these medications may contribute to antibiotic resistance or diminish the effectiveness of antivirals in the future. We can appreciate the value of antibiotics and antivirals in battling infections and utilizing them appropriately to promote better health if we grasp their purpose and functions.

The disparities between bacterial and viral infections, as well as the demand for specialized treatments.

When it comes to infections, it's vital to grasp the distinctions between bacterial and viral infections because they need different treatments.

Bacterial infections are created by microscopic organisms that can infect our bodies and cause disease. Urinary tract infections, strep throat, and bacterial pneumonia are all instances of bacterial ailments.

Bacterial infections typically produce fever, localized discomfort, and pus formation. Antibiotics, which are medications that are specifically designed to kill germs or inhibit their growth, can be used to treat them. Antibiotics operate by focusing on certain components of bacteria and limiting their capacity to survive and develop. To ensure thorough eradication of the germs, it is necessary to use antibiotics with prudence and complete the entire course as advised.

Virus Infections: Viruses are not the same as bacteria. They are quite small and cannot thrive on their own. Instead, they enter our cells and use them to multiply.

The common cold, flu, and viral hepatitis are all instances of viral infections. Coughing, sneezing, sore throat, and weariness are common symptoms of viral infections. Viruses, unlike bacteria, cannot be killed by antibiotics because their structures and functions are different.

Antiviral drugs, on the other hand, are designed to restrict viral reproduction, ease symptoms, and expedite recovery. Antivirals function by preventing the virus from replicating and spreading by targeting key processes in the viral life cycle. However, not all viral illnesses have specialized antiviral drugs, and supportive care is frequently the primary approach to treating symptoms and helping the immune system to fight the virus.

Understanding the distinctions between bacterial and viral infections is crucial because it allows healthcare providers to determine the most effective treatment.

Using medications to treat viral infections is ineffective and may lead to antibiotic resistance, an increasing global concern. Antivirals, on the other hand, primarily target viral infections and can be useful in some circumstances.

Drug-Resistant Bacteria and Viruses on the Rise

Discussing the evolution of drug-resistant bacteria and viruses, as well as the obstacles that these resistant species confront, as well as the limitations of classical antibiotics and antivirals.

There has been a substantial increase in the number of drug-resistant bacteria and viruses in recent years. This means that certain strains of bacteria and viruses have gained the ability to resist the effects of conventional antibiotics and antivirals that were previously successful against them.

Drug-Resistant Strains: Bacteria and viruses can adapt and change over time, resulting in the formation of drug-resistant strains.

This happens when these organisms undergo genetic modifications that make them less vulnerable to the treatments designed to target them. Abuse or overuse of antibiotics and antivirals, insufficient treatment regimens, and incorrect prescribing methods may all contribute to the creation and spread of drug-resistant strains.

Drug-Resistant Bacteria and Viruses: Drug-resistant bacteria and viruses offer substantial difficulties in healthcare. When these resistant germs create infections, it becomes more difficult to treat them adequately.

This can lead to longer sickness, increased healthcare expenses, a higher incidence of complications, and, in extreme situations, even death. Drug-resistant illnesses are becoming a rising international health concern due to limited treatment possibilities.

Limitations of Conventional Antibiotics and Antivirals: For many decades, conventional antibiotics and antivirals have been highly successful instruments in the fight against infections.

Their effectiveness, however, is being limited by the rise of drug-resistant forms. These medicines are meant to target specific mechanisms within bacteria or viruses; however, if those mechanisms alter due to resistance, the medications become less effective. Furthermore, typical antibiotics usually have a narrow spectrum of activity, which means they only operate against particular types of bacteria.

This narrow range of action contributes to the issues caused by drug-resistant microorganisms.

Addressing the problem of drug-resistant bacteria and viruses demands a diverse strategy. To address this global concern, initiatives such as responsible and proper use of antibiotics and antivirals, increased infection prevention and control techniques, the creation of novel pharmaceuticals, and research into alternative therapies such as natural herbs are being researched.

Chapter One: The Potential of Natural Herbs as Alternatives

Utilizing natural herbs as an alternative disease-fighting strategy.

Natural herbs have emerged as a viable alternative to mainstream pharmaceuticals in the fight against diseases. Let's look into the topic of natural herbs and their potential benefits:

Traditional Wisdom and Herbal Medicine: Throughout history, different cultures have depended on the medicinal capabilities of herbs to address a variety of health problems, including infections.

Traditional medicinal systems, such as Ayurveda, Traditional Chinese Medicine, and Indigenous healing methods, have long acknowledged natural plants' curative power. These herbs comprise bioactive chemicals with antimicrobial, antibacterial, antiviral, and immune-boosting activities.

Broader Spectrum of Activity: One of the benefits of natural herbs is their capacity to combat a wide spectrum of pathogens. Unlike conventional drugs, which usually target specific types of bacteria or viruses, many herbs have a broader range of activity.

This means they may be effective against a wide spectrum of bacteria or viruses, making them a versatile alternative in the fight against the disease.

Reduced Resistance: The rise of drug-resistant diseases has highlighted the need for innovative treatments. Natural herbs may give a therapeutic therapy by minimizing the risk of resistance development.

Herbs' complex variety of bioactive components can operate synergistically, making it more difficult for bacteria to acquire resistance as opposed to single-target drugs. This feature of herbs makes them a significant resource in the fight against disease.

Supporting the Immune System: Natural herbs, in addition to their direct antibacterial qualities, can also boost and expand the immune system. A strong immune response is vital in the battle against infections.

Some herbs contain immunomodulatory qualities, which means they can help regulate and improve the body's immunological function, increasing overall well-being and aiding in illness recovery.

Complementary and Integrative Approaches: It is crucial to recognize that using natural herbs as an alternate method does not necessarily imply entirely substituting conventional treatments.

Instead, they can be integrated into a holistic plan that encompasses the best of both worlds. Natural herbs can augment conventional treatments by boosting their effectiveness or reducing the dosage necessary.

However, the employment of natural plants must be done with prudence. Not all herbs are appropriate for every person or every type of ailment.

Herbal remedies should only be taken under the supervision of qualified healthcare professionals who can provide correct dosing instructions, research potential herb-drug interactions, and track the course of treatment.

The Advantages and Drawbacks of Natural Antibiotic and Antiviral Herbs

When applied as an alternative to conventional antibiotics and antivirals, natural herbs give several benefits. However, their limitations must be carefully addressed. Let's take a deeper look at these points:

Natural Antibiotic and Antiviral Herbs' Advantages:

Greater Effectiveness: Natural herbs contain a varied spectrum of bioactive components that have antibacterial capabilities. Herbs may have a greater spectrum of activity than conventional drugs, which frequently target specific types of germs or viruses. This means they may be effective against a wide range of bacterial strains or species. Herbs comprise a wide spectrum of compounds that can work together to boost their overall effectiveness in treating diseases.

Reduced Resistance Development: The creation of drug-resistant germs and viruses has become a major worry. One advantage of natural herbs is their capacity to lower the danger of resistance development.

Herbs may be more difficult to develop resistance to than drugs that target a specific pathway because they have a complex variety of bioactive components. Because of the lower danger of resistance, herbs are an intriguing alternative in the fight against infections.

Different Modes of Action: Natural herbs can exert their antibacterial qualities in a variety of ways. Some herbs may limit microbe development or reproduction, disrupt cell membranes, or interfere with metabolic activities. This comprehensive technique makes it more difficult for bacteria or viruses to adapt and acquire resistance as they must traverse several barriers.

Enhancing the Body's Defense Mechanisms: Natural herbs not only have antibacterial effects, but they also provide extra advantages by increasing the body's defense mechanisms.

They can improve immunological function, leading to a better immune response to infections. Some plants contain anti-inflammatory qualities, which can help to ease symptoms and reduce inflammation caused by illnesses. Herbs contribute to overall wellness and aid in the recovery process by reinforcing the body's natural defenses.

Natural Antibiotic and Antiviral Herbs' Limitations: Potency and Standardization: The potency and effectiveness of herbs may vary based on factors such as plant species, cultivation conditions, and preparation techniques. Standardization of herbal products can be difficult, resulting in differences in bioactive component concentration. For reliable outcomes, it is necessary to apply high-quality herbs and standardized herbal mixes.

While herbs have a long history of traditional use, scientific evidence supporting their effectiveness as antibiotics or antivirals is usually weak. More study is needed to understand the particular mechanisms of action, optimum doses, and potential pharmaceutical interactions.

It is vital to utilize herbs with prudence and to speak with healthcare specialists who are knowledgeable in herbal medicine.

Individual variances: Because of factors such as genetic differences, underlying health conditions, or concurrent drugs, each person may react differently to herbal therapy.

What works well for one individual may not work well for another. To ensure the safe and successful use of herbal medicines, individualized strategies, and professional guidance are required.

Natural herbs should be considered as a supplement to conventional medicine rather than a complete replacement.

In some circumstances, conventional drugs may be essential to treat serious or life-threatening conditions. Integrating herbs with conventional treatments under the guidance of healthcare professionals can create a more comprehensive and successful strategy for infection management.

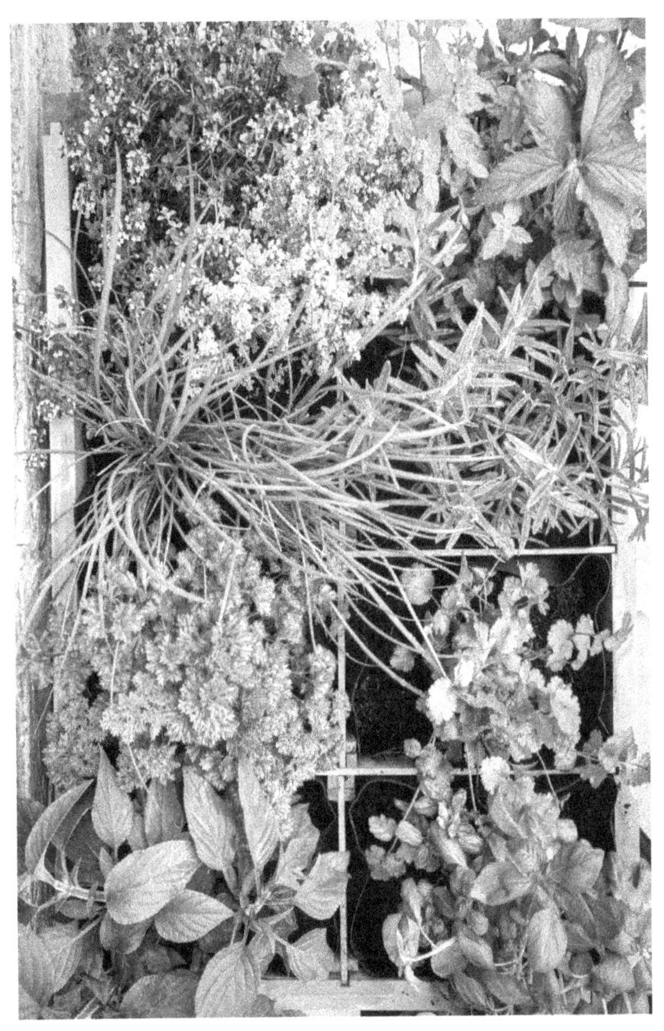

Chapter Two: Fundamental Herbal Medicine Concepts

Understanding the Action Mechanisms of Natural Antibiotic and Antiviral Herbs

This section introduces the methods of action of natural antibiotics and antiviral herbs. We examine how these herbs battle disease by attacking microbes such as bacteria and viruses. Understanding these pathways allows us to better understand how herbs function and how they can be used effectively in the battle against infections.

When we mention techniques of action, we are referring to the precise ways in which natural herbs kill germs. Let us break it down into simpler terms:

Overview of Mechanisms of Action: To begin, we will present a brief overview of the numerous methods by which natural herbs tackle disease. Directly limiting the development and reproduction of bacteria, changing their cell structures, interfering with their metabolic processes, stimulating the body's immune system, and regulating the inflammatory response are among the strategies used.

Microbial Growth and Reproduction Inhibition: Natural herbs have characteristics that can directly suppress microbial growth and reproduction. They prevent the spread and multiplication of dangerous germs and viruses in human bodies by doing so.

Disruption of Microbial Cell Structures: Another method natural herbs operate is by disrupting microbe cell structures. They impair the integrity of bacterial or viral cells, making survival and growth difficult.

Interference with Microbial Metabolic Processes: Natural herbs can impair bacterial metabolic processes. This means that they interrupt the regular functioning of bacteria or viruses, leading them to malfunction and eventually die.

Immune System Activation: Herbs can activate and improve the body's immune system, which is our natural protection against diseases. Herbs enable our bodies to fight against invading microorganisms by strengthening our immune response.

Regulation of Inflammatory Response: Inflammation is our bodies natural response to infections. However, severe inflammation can cause pain and tissue damage. Natural herbs can modulate this inflammatory response, lowering inflammation and related symptoms.

Synergistic Effects of Many Mechanisms: Natural herbs can sometimes work in tandem, employing many mechanisms of action at the same time. This synergistic impact boosts their overall efficacy in treating infections.

Factors Influencing Mechanisms of Action: A multitude of factors can affect how herbs function against germs. This covers the herb's species, the precise bioactive components present, and how they interact with bacteria or our bodies. These factors can alter the effectiveness of herbs in fighting infections.

Infection management: Understanding the mechanisms of action of natural herbs provides practical benefits in infection control. It helps healthcare practitioners and individuals to make informed decisions regarding the use of herbs and to examine their potential in various infection treatment strategies.

We acquire valuable insights into how natural herbs fight diseases by knowing their mechanisms of action. This information can lead to the successful use of herbs and the development of specialized therapies for certain illnesses.

Understanding how natural antibiotics and antiviral herbs act to fight disease

Understanding how natural antibiotics and antiviral herbs function to fight infections is crucial to optimizing their health benefits. Let us break it down into simpler terms:

Natural Antibiotic and Antiviral Herbs: These are herbs that have been proven to have antibacterial and antiviral properties.

Natural herbs, as opposed to manufactured antibiotics and antivirals, are generated from plants and have been used in traditional medicine for millennia.

Infection Control: When our bodies are exposed to dangerous germs like bacteria or viruses, they can cause infections and make us unwell. Natural herbs have unique qualities that allow them to target and treat specific ailments.

Natural herbs offer a range of techniques to combat disease. They have the power to directly block bacterial growth and reproduction, destroy cell structures, interfere with metabolic activities, stimulate the immune system, and regulate the body's inflammatory response.

Natural herbs include components that can directly block the growth and reproduction of germs or viruses. This inhibits bacteria from replicating and spreading in our bodies.

Cell architecture disruption: Certain herbs can influence the design of bacterial or viral cells, affecting their integrity. This makes it more difficult for bacteria to thrive and grow, eventually leading to extinction.

Interference with Bacterial Metabolic Activities: Natural herbs can interfere with bacterial metabolic activities. Herbs impede the ability of bacteria or viruses to function correctly by interfering with these processes, resulting in their mortality.

Immune System Activation: Herbs can also be used to activate and boost our immune systems. This implies they enhance our bodies' natural defense processes in recognizing and destroying invading bacteria.

Inflammatory response regulation: Infections typically result in inflammation as an immune system response. Natural herbs can aid in the management of this inflammatory response, lowering excessive inflammation and accompanying symptoms.

We can make informed decisions about the use of natural antibiotics and antiviral herbs in maintaining health and controlling illnesses if we understand how they operate to combat infections.

They give a natural, supposedly safer alternative to antibiotics and antivirals. However, it is vital to consult with healthcare professionals for suitable aid and to assure the correct infection diagnosis and treatment.

Investigating the diverse antibacterial properties of natural plants

Exploring the numerous antimicrobial features presented by natural herbs involves knowing how these herbs possess properties that can aid in the war against germs such as bacteria and viruses.

Antimicrobial Properties: Antimicrobial properties refer to a substance's ability to suppress or remove the growth of germs, in this case, natural herbs. Herbs with these qualities can treat diseases caused by bacteria, viruses, and other dangerous organisms.

Natural herbs are derived from plants and have been utilized for therapeutic purposes throughout history. They contain bioactive compounds, which contribute to their antibacterial activities.

Microorganism Types: Microorganisms comprise a wide spectrum of microscopic organisms such as bacteria, viruses, fungi, and parasites. Different herbs have varying degrees of potency against different types of bacteria.

Microbial Growth Inhibition: Natural herbs can reduce germ growth by reducing reproduction and proliferation. This helps to keep harmful bacteria and viruses at bay in our bodies.

Microbial Killing: Certain herbs can directly kill microorganisms, resulting in their removal. This is especially useful in the treatment of illnesses caused by harmful bacteria or viruses.

Broad-Spectrum Activity: Some herbs have broad-spectrum activity, which implies they are effective against a wide variety of bacteria. Because of their versatility, they are useful in addressing a wide range of disorders.

Specificity: On the other hand, some herbs may have particular antibacterial qualities, allowing them to target specific types of microbes more efficiently. This differentiation offers specific treatment choices for certain illnesses.

Natural herbs contain bioactive components such as phenols, flavonoids, alkaloids, and essential oils, which contribute to their antibacterial capabilities. These substances can disrupt microbial processes, impair cell structures, and inhibit microbial growth.

Understanding how natural herbs directly suppress germ growth

Understanding how natural herbs directly suppress germ growth and reproduction is crucial to understanding their effectiveness in combating ailments. Let us break it down into simpler terms:

Microorganism Growth and Reproduction: Microorganisms, such as bacteria and viruses, can multiply rapidly in human systems, causing sickness and illness. Controlling and treating these illnesses includes preventing their development and reproduction.

Direct Inhibition: Certain natural herbs have qualities that allow them to directly inhibit germ growth and reproduction.

Replication Interference: Herbs can interfere with microorganism replication. Herbs' ability to reproduce is impeded by the targeting of crucial components or processes required for replication.

Disrupting Cellular Structures: Certain herbs can disturb the structures of microorganisms, affecting their integrity and hampering their ability to function efficiently. This disturbance weakens the germs and prevents them from successfully replicating.

Certain herbs possess bioactive chemicals that can target enzymes or proteins necessary for microbial growth and reproduction. Herbs decrease bacteria's capacity to survive and proliferate by blocking certain enzymes or proteins.

Nutrient Blocking: Microorganisms require nutrients to grow and multiply. Some herbs have components that can inhibit bacteria from getting these critical nutrients, depriving them of the resources they require to survive.

Natural herbs may include components that may cause damage to bacteria' genetic material (DNA/RNA). This damage can hamper their capacity to replicate effectively, eventually leading to extinction.

Cell Wall Disruption: Bacterial cells have a protective outer layer known as the cell wall. Certain herbs can decrease cell wall formation, weakening bacteria and making them more vulnerable to immune responses or other antimicrobial effects.

This knowledge helps us to select relevant herbs for specific types of infections and build effective treatment programs. However, it is crucial to note that the efficacy of herbs varies, and contacting healthcare specialists is recommended for correct diagnosis and guidance in utilizing herbal remedies.

Investigate Natural Herbs

It is vital to understand how natural herbs might disrupt the cell structures of bacteria and viruses to limit the survival and multiplication of these hazardous diseases.

Bacterial and viral cell structures: Bacteria and viruses have a range of cell structures that play a key role in their survival and ability to cause illness.

Disrupting Cell Structures: Certain natural herbs have qualities that allow them to disrupt the cell structures of bacteria and viruses.

Bacterial Cell Weakening: Some herbs possess components that can weaken the outer structures of bacterial cells. This degeneration impairs the integrity of the cells, making it difficult for them to live and function effectively.

Improving Viral Replication: Viruses replicate and multiply in host cells. Certain herbs can affect the viral replication process by changing the viral cell structures involved. Herbs help to limit the spread of viral infections by reducing viral replication.

Cell Membranes as a Target: Cell membranes are the protective outer coverings of bacteria and viruses. Natural herbs may have bioactive substances that interact with and disturb these cell membranes, leading them to become unstable.

Interfering with Important Functions: By targeting specific components within bacteria and viruses' cell structures, natural herbs can impair vital functions. This interference affects their ability to complete critical processes required for life and replication.

Increasing Vulnerability: Herbs make bacteria and viruses more vulnerable to other antimicrobial actions, such as immunological responses or the effects of other herbal chemicals, by changing cell structures.

Limiting Spread and Multiplication: Herbs help restrict the spread and multiplication of bacteria and viruses in human bodies by inhibiting their survival and replication through the destruction of cell components. This aids in the treatment and management of disorders.

Investigating how natural herbs can interfere with microbial metabolic processes requires knowing how these herbs might disturb important chemical events within bacteria, decreasing their ability to work properly.

Microbial Metabolic Processes: Microorganisms, such as bacteria and viruses, rely on a range of metabolic processes to obtain energy, develop, and carry out vital functions.

Interference with Metabolic Activities: Natural herbs offer qualities that allow them to interfere with microorganism metabolic activities.

Key Metabolic routes: Microorganisms have particular metabolic routes that are engaged in processes including energy production, food intake, and chemical synthesis. These pathways could be possible targets for herb action.

Enzyme Disruption: Herbs can have bioactive chemicals that interact with enzymes found in bacteria. Enzymes play key roles in metabolic reactions, and interfering with them impairs the germs' capacity to function properly.

Energy generation inhibition: Natural herbs may block the creation of energy molecules such as ATP within bacteria. This shortage of energy weakens the bacteria and affects their capacity to develop and execute critical jobs.

Improving Nutrient Uptake: Some herbs can interfere with microbes' uptake and usage of nutrients. This nutritional shortage deprives the bacteria of the resources they require to continue growing and living.

Disrupting manufacturing processes: Microorganisms rely on the manufacture of many substances, such as proteins and nucleic acids, to function properly. Certain herbs can interfere with these synthesis processes, limiting microorganisms' ability to function properly.

Overall Impairment: Herbs hinder the proper functioning of microbes by interfering with microbial metabolic pathways, limiting their ability to live, grow, and cause harm.

We can obtain insight into natural herbs' antimicrobial action by knowing how they can interfere with bacteria's metabolic activities. This knowledge enables us to select relevant herbs for treating specific types of infections and design successful treatment procedures.

How many natural herbs affect the immune system?

Studying how natural herbs can alter the immune system to increase the body's defenses against infections includes studying their potential to change and strengthen our immunological response. Infections and the Immune System: The immune system is the body's defense mechanism against pathogens such as bacteria, viruses, and other organisms that can cause infections.

Natural herbs have qualities that can affect or regulate the immune system, modifying its activity and improving the body's resistance to illnesses.

Immune Response: When the body discovers pathogens, the immune system mounts an attack to remove them. This reaction involves a variety of immune cells, including white blood cells and antibodies, as well as chemical messengers known as cytokines.

Immune boosting: Certain herbs include bioactive components that can improve immune cell function and create a stronger immunological response. This can involve enhancing the activity and creation of immune cells, as well as their ability to recognize and attack infections.

Antibacterial Activity: Natural herbs can help boost immune cells' antibacterial activity. This can include raising antibody production or increasing the activity of phagocytes, which are immune cells that eat and remove infections.

Immune Response Balancing: To work effectively, the immune system must be carefully balanced. Some herbs possess characteristics that assist modulate the immune response, preventing it from becoming overactive or producing excessive inflammation.

Anti-inflammatory Effects: Inflammation is a natural immune system response, but excessive inflammation can be damaging. Certain herbs have anti-inflammatory characteristics that can aid in the decrease of inflammation and the promotion of a healthy immune response.

Supporting Overall Immune Health: Natural herbs can also supply crucial nutrients and antioxidants that enhance overall immune health. A strong immune system is more able to ward off infections and sustain overall health.

Investigating how natural herbs can activate immune cells, such as macrophages and natural killer cells, to boost their antimicrobial activity requires investigating how these herbs can stimulate specific immune cells to fight infections more effectively.

Infections and Immune Cells: Immune cells, particularly macrophages and natural killer cells, play key roles in the body's defense against infections. They are in charge of detecting and removing infections.

Immune Cell Activation: Certain natural herbs have characteristics that can activate specific immune cells, boosting their antibacterial impact.

Macrophages are immune cells that absorb and kill infections. Certain herbs can activate macrophages, enhancing their activity and ability to destroy invading infections.

Natural killer cells are immune cells that specialize in finding and killing contaminated cells or cancer cells. Some herbs can stimulate natural killer cells, enhancing their activity in combating disease.

Increasing antibacterial activity: Natural herbs activate immune cells, which promotes antibacterial activity.

This can involve enhanced pathogen detection and targeting, as well as more powerful killing mechanisms to eradicate the invaders.

Increasing Immunological Response: Herbs can increase the overall immunological response to infections by activating immune cells. This can result in a more powerful defensive system and enhanced control of microbial dangers.

Supporting the Immune System: Natural herbs can give the required components and chemicals to help immune cells function efficiently. This comprises giving vital nutrients and antioxidants to help immune cells retain their health and activity.

Immune Cell Activation: Herbs that activate immune cells help to maintain a healthy immunological response. It contributes to ensuring that immune cells are properly stimulated without producing excessive inflammation or immune system instability.

Researching how natural herbs can assist manage the body's inflammatory response demands researching their capacity to control and lessen excessive inflammation that can occur during infections.

Infections and the Inflammatory Reaction: When the body identifies an infection, it launches an inflammatory reaction as a defense tactic. Inflammation aids in the elimination of infections and promotes recovery.

Regulating Inflammation: Natural herbs have qualities that can aid in the regulation of the body's inflammatory response, keeping it from becoming excessive or detrimental.

Excessive Inflammation: Excessive inflammation can arise as a result of the immune system's response to an infection. This elevated inflammation could cause tissue damage and other concerns.

Anti-inflammatory properties: Certain plants possess anti-inflammatory chemicals. These substances can aid in the reduction of inflammation and the restoration of the body's immunological equilibrium.

Inhibiting Inflammatory Mediators: Bioactive components in natural herbs may inhibit the synthesis or activity of inflammatory mediators such as cytokines and prostaglandins. This inhibition helps to minimize inflammation and its harmful effects.

Immune Reaction Balancing: Herbs can help maintain a healthy immune system by lowering the inflammatory reaction. This balance ensures that inflammation is adequately managed and focused to attack the infection without causing unnecessary harm to healthy tissues.

Symptom Relief: Excessive inflammation can cause symptoms such as pain, edema, and fever. Herbs can help ease these symptoms by lowering inflammation, offering relief, and increasing overall well-being during infections.

Supporting the Healing Process: In addition to decreasing inflammation, herbs may have qualities that aid in the healing process. This can involve stimulating tissue repair and regeneration, which can aid in infection recovery.

Understanding how specific herbs, when used together, might increase each other's antimicrobial and immune-modulating characteristics is one way to emphasize the possible synergistic effects of mixing diverse herbs.

Synergistic Effects: Synergy is defined as the combined effect of numerous factors that are greater than the sum of their separate effects. When it comes to herbs, specific mixtures can have synergistic advantages.

Antimicrobial characteristics: Many herbs possess natural chemicals with antimicrobial qualities, which means they can prevent the growth and activity of microorganisms such as bacteria and viruses.

Immune-Modulating qualities: Some herbs have immune-modulating qualities, which means they can affect and regulate the immune system's response, enhancing its ability to fight infections.

When certain herbs are combined, their antibacterial and immune-modulating characteristics can function together in a complimentary manner, resulting in a more strong and effective response to infections.

Increasing antibacterial activity: Combining herbs may result in a larger spectrum of antibacterial activity. Different herbs may target different types of germs or have distinct modes of action, providing a comprehensive strategy for sickness prevention.

Immunological Response Enhancement: The combination of herbs can also synergistically improve the immunological response. The combination of herbs can function together to maximize the body's defense capacity by influencing various components of the immune system, such as increasing immune cells or regulating inflammatory processes.

Potentiating Effects: Some herbs may include chemicals that boost the absorption or activity of other herbs when combined. This can boost their antibacterial and immune-modulating activities.

Personalized Combinations: The particular mix of herbs and their ratios may alter depending on the desired purpose and individual requirements. Herbalists and healthcare specialists can assist in finding the optimum combinations based on the pathogens being targeted and the individual's health situation.

Understanding the potential synergistic effects of combining different herbs exposes the possibility of increasing their antibacterial and immune-modulating characteristics. It is crucial to highlight, however, that herbal combinations should be taken with caution and under the guidance of qualified practitioners.

Examining several factors that can impact the efficiency of natural herbs as antibiotics and antivirals

Examining several factors that can impact the efficiency of natural herbs as antibiotics and antivirals involves an examination of several aspects that can influence how well these herbs perform in battling infections.

Herb Selection: The selection of herbs used as antibiotics and antivirals has a considerable impact on their efficacy. Because different herbs have variable degrees of antibacterial and antiviral action, picking the correct herbs for certain illnesses is crucial.

Quality and Purity: The quality and purity of the herbs utilized can have a considerable impact on their performance. To ensure the efficacy and safety of the herbs, they must be obtained from trusted sources and go through proper quality control techniques.

Plant portion and preparation: The exact portion of the plant used (such as leaves, roots, or flowers) as well as the method of preparation (such as teas, tinctures, or extracts) may influence the concentration and availability of bioactive chemicals responsible for antibacterial and antiviral effects.

Dosage and Administration: For herbal remedies to be successful, exact dosage and administration are essential. The correct dosage must be determined depending on the individual's age, weight, and health situation to ensure the herbs are taken safely and successfully.

Synergy with other medicines: Natural herbs can be used in conjunction with standard medical therapy to boost their efficacy. Understanding how herbs interact with various medications or therapies is crucial for assuring compatibility and limiting any potential unwanted effects.

Individual Differences: The results of herbal therapies can differ from person to person. Herbs' effectiveness as antibiotics and antivirals can be modified by factors such as inheritance, overall health, and underlying illnesses. Personalized tactics that address individual characteristics are crucial for attaining the greatest results.

Administration Time: The timing of herbal administration can alter its effectiveness. Herbs may be more beneficial in some circumstances when supplied during specific stages of infection or when taken preventively to improve the immune system.

Adherence to Suggested Protocols: It is vital for the success of herbal medicines to follow established protocols and guidelines. It is vital to speak with trained healthcare practitioners or herbalists who can advise on the dosage, frequency, and duration of herbal therapy.

By investigating these distinct qualities, we can acquire a better knowledge of how they influence the efficiency of natural herbs such as antibiotics and antivirals.

For efficient infection management, it is necessary to approach herbal medicines with prudence, consult healthcare specialists or herbalists, and blend them with conventional medical care.

It is vital to understand the value of using high-quality herbs and standardized herbal products to maintain constant potency and effectiveness. Let us break it down into simpler terms:

Quality of Herbs: The quality of herbs used in herbal products could vary substantially. Herbs of high quality are sourced from recognized vendors and submitted to extensive quality control procedures to assure their purity, authenticity, and potency.

High-quality herbs have consistent levels of bioactive chemicals, which are responsible for their therapeutic qualities. This consistency ensures that each batch of herbal medications consistently produces the required therapeutic effects.

Standardization is a method that guarantees the herbal product includes a standardized amount or concentration of key active components. This procedure offers the herbal product's potency and effectiveness more control.

Reliable Results: Using standardized herbal remedies means that the desired therapeutic benefits are frequently attained. This consistency is especially crucial when employing herbs such as antibiotics and antivirals, as consistent potency is critical for optimal efficacy.

Considerations for Safety: High-quality and standardized herbal products are more likely to go through rigorous safety testing to ensure they are devoid of toxins, heavy metals, and hazardous compounds. This feature is crucial for assuring the safety of those who consume herbal goods.

Choosing herbal medicines from known and trusted brands or manufacturers boosts the possibility of acquiring high-quality and standardized products. It is advisable to explore and choose products with a solid reputation and that meet quality criteria.

Seeking professional advice from experienced healthcare professionals, herbalists, or herbal medicine experts can help assure the selection of high-quality herbs and standardized herbal products.

Based on their knowledge and experience, these professionals can make advice.

Quality Assurance: Choosing herbal products made in facilities that conform to good manufacturing principles (GMP) gives an added layer of quality assurance. GMP ensures that herbal items are manufactured in a consistent and controlled manner. Exploring the ideal dosage and duration of treatment with natural herbs is crucial for effective infection management.

Dosage: The dosage is the amount of herbal product or herb that should be eaten to treat a specific infection. The correct dosage is established by examining criteria such as the individual's age, weight, overall health, and the severity of the infection.

Herbs have a therapeutic range, which suggests that there is a precise dosage range where they are most effective and safe. It is crucial to keep within this range to optimize the benefits and reduce the chance of side effects.

Individual Variations: Because of variances in metabolism, sensitivity, and underlying health issues, the appropriate dosage may change between individuals. What works for one individual might not work for another. As a result, it is vital to take into consideration individual variances and consult with healthcare specialists or herbalists for precise dosage recommendations.

Treatment Duration: The treatment duration refers to how long herbal remedies should be administered to effectively manage an infection. Some infections may require merely short-term treatment, while others may necessitate longer-term or intermittent herbal use.

Acute vs. Chronic Infections: Treatment time varies depending on whether the infection is acute (short-term) or chronic (long-term). Acute infections may require less time to treat, whereas chronic infections may necessitate more time.

Follow guidelines: It is vital to stick to the dosage and treatment time guidelines offered by healthcare professionals or herbalists. Deviating from the specified guidelines may result in substandard outcomes or major hazards.

Monitoring Progress: It is crucial to determine the success of herbal treatment by routinely checking symptoms and progress. If there is no improvement or the situation worsens, it is vital to seek medical assistance as soon as possible.

Precautions: While herbs are generally regarded safe, it is vital to be mindful of potential interactions with other drugs or underlying health conditions. To ensure the safe and efficient use of herbal treatments, inform healthcare practitioners about any ongoing therapy or health concerns.

Individuals can increase the efficacy of herbal remedies for healing ailments by researching the appropriate dosage and treatment time for natural herbs. Seeking aid from medical doctors or herbalists.

Recognizing the necessity of evaluating individual differences in response to herbal therapies includes acknowledging that different persons may respond differently to herbal remedies.

Genetic Factors: Our genetic makeup can have an impact on how our systems absorb and respond to herbal medications. Genetic variances can affect how rapidly we absorb herbs, how our immune system reacts to them, and our overall vulnerability to specific treatments. Understanding these genetic features can aid in the tailoring of herbal medicines for increased efficacy.

Individual health concerns have a huge impact on how the body responds to herbal medications.

Existing medical disorders, such as liver or renal illness, may impede the body's capacity to digest herbal components.

To ensure safe and effective use, it is necessary to assess these illnesses and their potential interactions with herbal therapies.

Concurrent prescriptions: If a person is taking other prescriptions in addition to herbal therapies, there is a possibility of drug interactions. Some plants can interact with prescription or over-the-counter pharmaceuticals, changing their effectiveness or creating unpleasant side effects.

It is vital to inform healthcare experts about any medications being used to verify compatibility and prevent dangers.

Allergies and Sensitivities: Some people are allergic or sensitive to specific plants or their compounds. To prevent unpleasant reactions, it is vital to be aware of any known allergies or sensitivities. If there is any question, allergy testing or contact with healthcare professionals could assist uncover potential risks.

Recognizing individual variances underscores the necessity of a tailored approach to herbal medications. Healthcare professionals or herbalists can examine an individual's unique traits, such as genetic factors, health issues, and concurrent medications, and create herbal therapies accordingly. This tailored strategy raises the likelihood of exceptional outcomes while eliminating potential hazards.

It is vital to address safety concerns while using natural herbs and to research potential interactions between herbal treatments and conventional drugs to ensure safe and effective therapy.

Natural herbs are typically considered harmless, yet it is vital to be informed of any hazards and safety practices. Some herbs can be dangerous if ingested in excessive quantities or for an extended period. It is vital to research and appreciates the potential hazards linked with various herbs before utilizing them.

Quality and Purity: The safety of herbal products needs to assure their quality and purity. Choosing renowned brands or sources that comply with quality standards such as Good Manufacturing Practices (GMP) decreases the danger of contamination or adulteration.

Individuals could develop allergies or sensitivities to numerous plants, just as they can to any other substance. To detect potential allergens, it is vital to be aware of any known allergies or sensitivities and to carefully read product labels.

Interactions with medications: Herbal remedies can interact with pharmaceuticals, either augmenting or lowering their effects. These interactions can have an impact on both the safety and efficacy of the herbal treatment and the drug. It is vital to contact healthcare specialists or pharmacists to find probable interactions and avert any bad outcomes.

Communicating with Healthcare specialists: It is vital to openly discuss the usage of herbal treatments with healthcare experts. They can offer vital insights into potential interactions with conventional pharmaceuticals as well as recommendations on safe and acceptable herbal use.

Medication Modifications: Depending on the conditions, healthcare practitioners may need to adjust the dosage or timing of conventional prescriptions when herbal medicines are used concurrently. This guarantees that the pharmaceuticals and plants function together safely and effectively.

Comprehensive Medication List: It is vital to preserve an up-to-date list of all drugs, including herbal therapies. This list should be shared with healthcare providers to guarantee accurate and full assessment and management information.

Monitoring and Reporting: It is vital to monitor for any harmful effects or changes in symptoms when utilizing herbal medicines. If any concerning symptoms arise, they must be reported immediately to healthcare specialists.

By addressing safety considerations when using natural herbs and discussing potential interactions with conventional drugs, consumers can avoid hazards and ensure safe and successful treatment. Researching herbs, buying high-quality goods, and being mindful of allergies.

Chapter Three: Common Antibacterial Herbs

Common antibacterial herbs are natural plant-based

Medicines that exhibit properties that can limit the growth and spread of bacteria. These plants have been exploited for years in traditional therapeutic approaches due to their antibacterial characteristics. Let's study some more deeply on some typical antibacterial herbs:

Garlic (Allium sativum): Garlic is famous for its excellent antibacterial characteristics. It contains compounds such as allicin that have exhibited antibacterial activity against a wide spectrum of bacteria, including both Gram-positive and Gram-negative strains.

Garlic can be consumed raw, cooked, or as a supplement to boost overall health and prevent bacterial diseases.

Ginger (Zingiber officinale): Ginger is not only recognized for its culinary purposes but also its antibacterial capabilities. It contains gingerol and shogaol compounds that give antimicrobial properties.

Ginger can be drunk as tea, added to dishes, or taken as a supplement to help digestion and treat bacterial infections.

Turmeric (Curcuma longa): Turmeric is a beautiful yellow spice often used in culinary and traditional medicine. It contains curcumin, a powerful chemical with antimicrobial actions.

Turmeric can be swallowed as a spice in cooking, brewed as tea, or taken as a supplement to boost immunological health and fight bacterial infections.

Oregano (Origanum vulgare): Oregano is a culinary

herb that also exhibits excellent antibacterial capabilities.

It contains compounds such as carvacrol and thymol that have been proven to limit the growth of certain bacteria. Oregano can be used as a dried herb in cooking, infused into oils, or taken as a supplement to support respiratory health and prevent bacterial infections.

Thyme (Thymus vulgaris): Thyme is an aromatic herb often used in cooking and herbal medicine. It contains thymol, a substance noted for its antimicrobial activities. Thyme can be used as a dried herb in cooking, brewed as a tea, or taken as a supplement to boost respiratory health and battle bacterial infections.

Echinacea (Echinacea purpurea): Echinacea is a well-known herb used to strengthen the immune system. It possesses antimicrobial characteristics that can help treat bacterial infections, particularly in the respiratory system. Echinacea is typically taken as a tea or used as a supplement to boost immune function.

Goldenseal (Hydrastis canadensis): Goldenseal is a perennial herb native to North America. It contains berberine, a chemical noted for its broad-spectrum antibacterial activity. Goldenseal is often utilized as a natural remedy for numerous ailments, notably bacterial infections.

Tea Tree Oil (Melaleuca alternifolia): Tea tree oil is derived from the leaves of the tea tree plant and is widely famous for its antibacterial capabilities.

It contains terpenes such as terpinene-4-ol, which have antibacterial effects against diverse pathogens. Tea tree oil can be used topically as a diluted solution to treat skin infections and wounds.

When utilizing these conventional antibacterial herbs, it is vital to consider individual sensitivities, allergies, and potential interactions with medicines. It is advisable to consult with healthcare specialists or herbalists for precise counsel on a dose, preparation techniques, and any side effects.

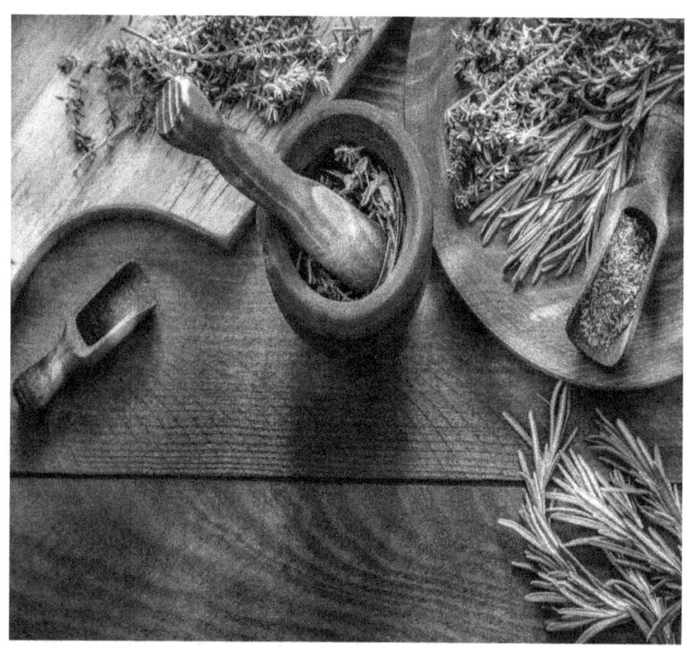

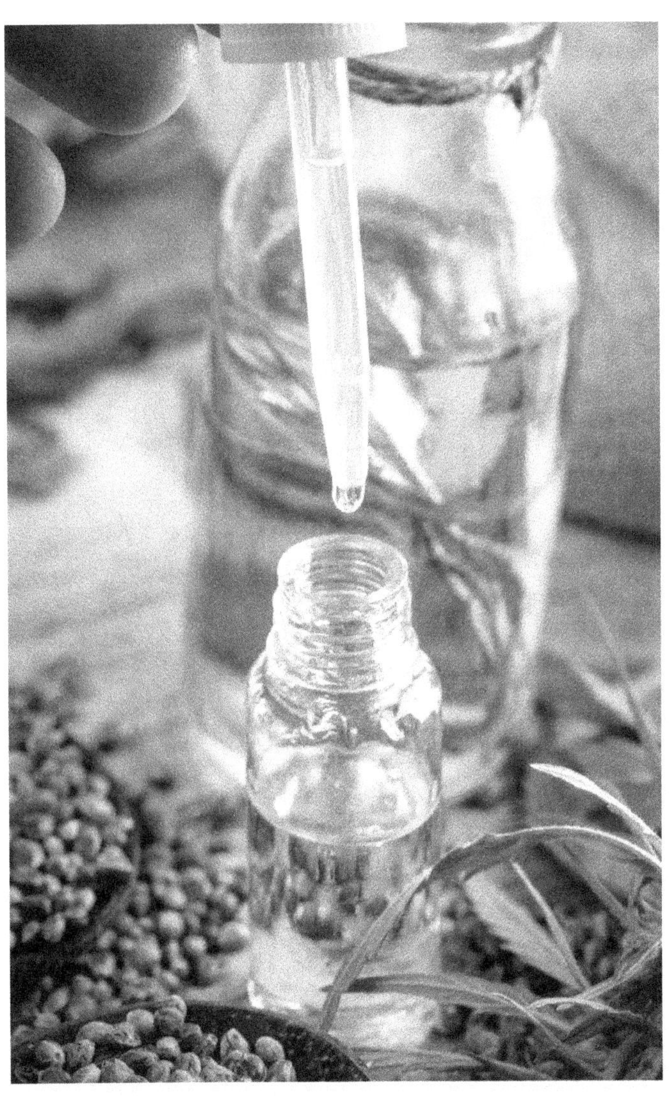

Chapter Four: Potent Antiviral Herbs

Potent antiviral herbs are natural plants that feature properties that can inhibit the multiplication and spread of viruses in the body.

These herbs have been traditionally used to stimulate the immune system and assist combat viral illnesses. Here are three extensively explained effective antiviral herbs:

Elderberry (Sambucus nigra): Elderberry is a well-known antiviral herb that has been used for millennia to treat viral infections, including the flu and common cold.

It comprises flavonoids and anthocyanins that help reduce viral replication and lower the severity and duration of viral symptoms. Elderberry can be consumed as a syrup, extract, or tea.

Echinacea (Echinacea purpurea): Echinacea, as noted before, is not only excellent for bacterial infections but also includes antiviral qualities. It can assist boost the immune system and enhance the body's natural resistance against illnesses. Echinacea is commonly administered as a tea, tincture, or supplement.

Astragalus (Astragalus membranaceous): Astragalus is a strong plant in traditional Chinese medicine recognized for its immune-boosting and antiviral capabilities. It enhances the body's resilience against viral infections and helps lessen the intensity of symptoms. Astragalus can be drunk as a tea or taken as a supplement.

Lemon Balm (Melissa officinalis): Lemon balm is a calming plant with antiviral effects, especially against herpes viruses. It contains compounds such as rosmarinic acid that decrease viral replication and provide treatment for cold sores and other viral infections. Lemon balm can be used as a tea, essential oil, or topical ointment.

Licorice Root (Glycyrrhiza glabra): Licorice root offers antiviral and immune-stimulating properties. It contains glycyrrhizin, which has been proven to limit the growth of certain viruses. Licorice root can be eaten as tea, decoction, or in the form of herbal supplements.

Olive Leaf (Olea europaea): Olive leaf extract has substantial antiviral effects, largely attributable to its active component named oleuropein. It has been discovered to restrict the reproduction of viruses and strengthen the immune system. Olive leaf extract is available in supplement form.

Ginger (Zingiber officinale): Ginger, famous for its immune-boosting benefits, also displays antiviral action. It can help fight against certain viruses and provide relief from symptoms connected with respiratory infections. Ginger can be ingested as tea, added to dishes, or taken as a supplement.

Andrographis (Andrographis paniculata): Andrographis is a herb commonly used in traditional Ayurvedic and Chinese medicine for its antiviral and immune-stimulating characteristics. It can help lower the intensity and duration of viral infections, especially respiratory tract infections. Andrographis is available in capsule or tablet form. When utilizing these potent antiviral herbs, it's vital to follow proper dosage guidelines and communication with healthcare providers, especially if you have underlying health concerns or are taking other medications.

These herbs can be introduced into your regimen as teas, extracts, supplements, or topical applications to support your immune system and assist against viral infections.

Remember, while these antiviral herbs can be beneficial, they should not substitute medical advice or treatment. If you feel you have a viral infection, it's vital to receive adequate medical attention for the correct diagnosis and information on treatment choices.

Chapter Five: Herbal Combinations for Enhanced Efficacy

Herbal mixes for enhanced efficacy relate to the strategy of combining various herbs to maximize their therapeutic advantages and create synergistic effects.

By combining chosen plants with complementary traits, their distinct activities can be amplified, resulting in a more potent and effective herbal medication.

Here is a full description of herbal combinations for higher effectiveness:

Immune-Boosting Blend: This combination combines herbs known for their immune-boosting benefits, such as echinacea, astragalus, and ginger. Echinacea stimulates immune cell activity, astragalus enhances immunological function, and ginger provides anti-inflammatory and antioxidant aid.

Together, these herbs operate synergistically to boost the immune system and enhance its ability to fight off infections.

Respiratory Support Formula: This blend concentrates on herbs that support respiratory health and relieves congestion. It may include herbs like thyme, licorice root, and eucalyptus.

Thyme serves as an expectorant, licorice root calms the respiratory tract, and eucalyptus helps cleanse the airways. Together, these herbs can help minimize respiratory issues and support healthier breathing.

Antiviral Synergy: This combination combines herbs with potent antiviral effects, such as elderberry, lemon balm, and olive leaf. Elderberry reduces viral replication, lemon balm has an antiviral impact against herpes viruses, and olive leaf extract aids against various viruses.

By combining these herbs, the antiviral effects are boosted, enabling overall protection against viral illnesses.

Digestive Calming Blend: This mixture focuses on herbs that help digestive health and reduce discomfort. It may include herbs like chamomile, peppermint, and ginger.

Chamomile soothes the digestive system, peppermint lowers spasms, and ginger promotes digestion. Together, these herbs can help alleviate digestive issues and build a peaceful and healthy digestive system.

Stress-Relief Formula: This blend combines plants known for their soothing and stress-reducing benefits, such as lavender, lemon balm, and passionflower. Lavender promotes relaxation, lemon balm has soothing characteristics, and passionflower helps reduce anxiety.

When combined, these herbs provide a synergistic effect, helping to reduce stress levels and generate a sense of peace. When applying herbal combinations, it is vital to check the proper ratios and dosages of each plant to guarantee safety and effectiveness.

It is vital to chat with a professional herbalist or healthcare practitioner to identify the optimal combination and dose depending on individual needs and health circumstances.

Integrating Natural Herbs into Daily Life

Integrating natural herbs into daily life refers to the practice of bringing herbs into our routines and lifestyles to promote health and well-being.

It comprises using herbs in various forms, such as teas, tinctures, culinary components, or herbal supplements, to enjoy their advantages regularly. Here is a full description of how to incorporate natural herbs into daily life:

Culinary Delights: One of the easiest ways to bring herbs into your daily life is through cooking. Many herbs, such as basil, thyme, rosemary, and oregano, not only add taste to your food but also give health advantages.

Sprinkle fresh or dried herbs onto your foods, use them in marinades or sauces, or infuse them into oils or vinegar for added flavor and medicinal effects.

Herbal Teas & Infusions: Herbal teas are a wonderful way to appreciate the medicinal benefits of herbs. Experiment with different herbal combinations, such as chamomile for relaxation, peppermint for digestion, or nettle for energy.

You can create herbal teas using fresh or dried herbs, or opt for ready-made tea bags or loose-leaf blends. Sip on herbal teas throughout the day as a relaxing and nutritious beverage.

Herbal Supplements: If you want a more concentrated sort of herbal treatment, consider integrating herbal supplements into your practice. These are available in pill, tablet, or liquid form and deliver handy and standardized dosages of herbs. However, it's vital to get high-quality supplements from renowned producers and speak with a healthcare practitioner for precise counsel on dosage and compatibility.

DIY Herbal remedies: Another technique to integrate plants into your daily life is by constructing your herbal medicines. This could include manufacturing herbal salves, tinctures, or infused oils for topical treatment, or developing herbal combinations for specific health requirements. You can locate various resources and recipes online or speak with a herbalist for guidance on making safe and effective herbal remedies.

Herbal Self-Care Rituals: Incorporating herbs into your self-care practice can promote relaxation and well-being. Create a quiet ambiance by using herbal essential oils for aromatherapy or adding herbs to your bathwater for a soothing soak. Herbal face masks, herbal steam.

Other ways to experience the therapeutic advantages of herbs while caring for your body include inhalations and herbal foot soaks.

Mindful Herbal Practices: Practice attention and mindfulness when you use herbs in your daily life. Take note of how herbs make you feel and any changes in your body, mind, or overall well-being. Keep a diary to record the effects of different herbs and combinations, allowing you to personalize your herbal journey to your individual needs.

While herbs can give various benefits, it is crucial to take them appropriately and check with a healthcare practitioner, especially if you have any pre-existing health concerns, are pregnant or nursing, or are taking drugs that may interact with herbs. Also, be mindful of any allergies or sensitivities to specific plants.

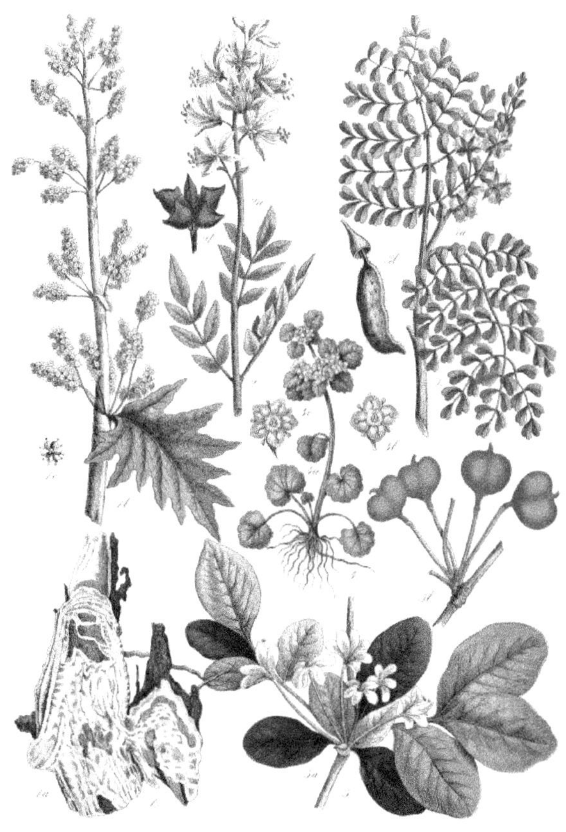

1. A. B. C., RHEUM PALMATUM, *Chinese Rhubarb*; – 2. A. B., DICTAMNUS ALBUS, *Burning Bush*;
3. A. B., CAESALPINIA BRASILIENSIS, *Caesalpinial*;
4. A. B. C., CHRYSOSPLENIUM ALTERNIFOLIUM, *Alternate-leaved Golden-saxifrage*;
5. A. B., GUAIACUM OFFICINALE, *Roughbark*

Chapter Six: Precautions and Adverse Reactions

When harnessing natural plants for their therapeutic potential, precautions, and side effects are significant problems. While herbs can provide various health advantages, it is vital to be aware of potential hazards and take steps to ensure safe and effective use.

Here is a full review of the risks and side effects of taking natural herbs:

Allergic Reactions: Certain herbs may induce allergic reactions in some persons. It is vital to be aware of any known sensitivities and to avoid plants that could trigger an allergic reaction.

Redness, itching, swelling, difficulty breathing, or gastrointestinal difficulties are frequent symptoms of an allergic reaction. If you suffer any allergic reactions after consuming a plant, discontinue using it and seek medical attention if necessary.

Interactions with drugs: Certain herbs can interact with medicines, including prescriptions, over-the-counter medications, and supplements. These interactions can affect the effectiveness of the herb or worsen its harmful effects.

It is vital to speak with a healthcare expert or pharmacist to establish whether there are any potential conflicts between herbs and your existing drugs.

Pregnancy and breast-feeding: When utilizing herbs during pregnancy and lactation, particular caution should be utilized. Some herbs may have harmful impacts on pregnancy or breastfeeding results. Before utilizing any herbs during these periods, contact a healthcare practitioner to guarantee the safety of both the mother and the infant.

Pre-existing Health Conditions: If you have pre-existing health conditions, you should carefully assess how certain herbs may affect your situation.

Some herbs may interfere with specific medical problems or drugs used to treat those disorders.

If you have any chronic or underlying health concerns, always consult with a healthcare practitioner before utilizing herbs.

Herb Quality and Contamination: Herb quality is crucial for their safety and effectiveness. It is vital to purchase herbs from recognized vendors who adhere to good production processes.

This helps ensure that the herbs are free of pollutants including pesticides, heavy metals, and microbiological infections. Look for herbal treatments that have been standardized to ensure consistent strength and quality.

Dosage and Duration: The optimal dosage and duration of herb use are crucial for safe and successful effects. It is vital to follow prescribed dose guidelines offered by trustworthy sources or healthcare specialists.

Extending the recommended dosage may result in unpleasant side effects. Furthermore, eating herbs for extended periods without pauses or beyond the approved duration may increase the chance of adverse repercussions.

Individual Variations: Because of their varied physiology, genetic traits, and overall health, each person may react differently to herbs. What works for one individual might not work for another.

It's crucial to pay attention to your body's reaction to herbs and make adjustments as needed. Begin with low doses and gradually increase as needed, keeping a watchful eye on any changes or unpleasant effects.

Hazardous Effects: While herbs are typically regarded as safe, they can have detrimental effects on some persons. Side effects could vary based on the plant and the individual. Common adverse effects include stomach pain, allergic reactions, sleepiness, and drug interactions. If you notice any concerned side effects, discontinue the use of the herb and check with a healthcare practitioner.

When using natural plants for medical purposes, it is necessary to take measures and be aware of possible harmful effects.

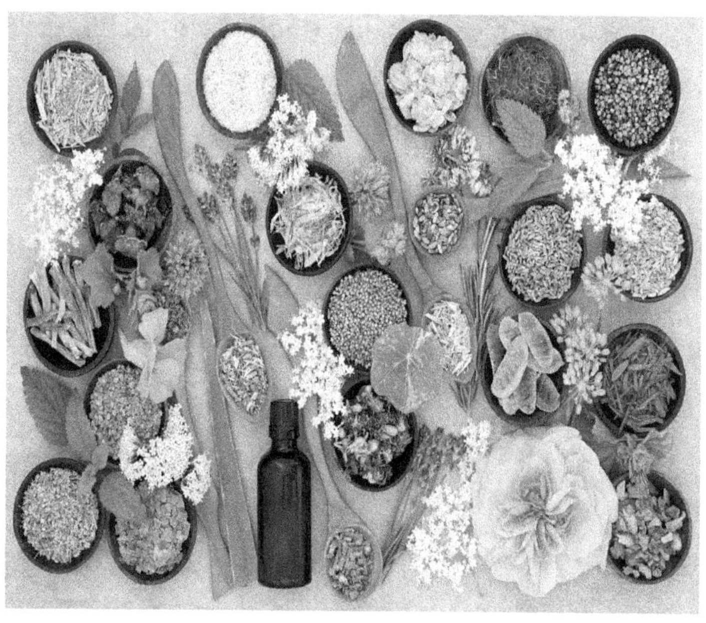

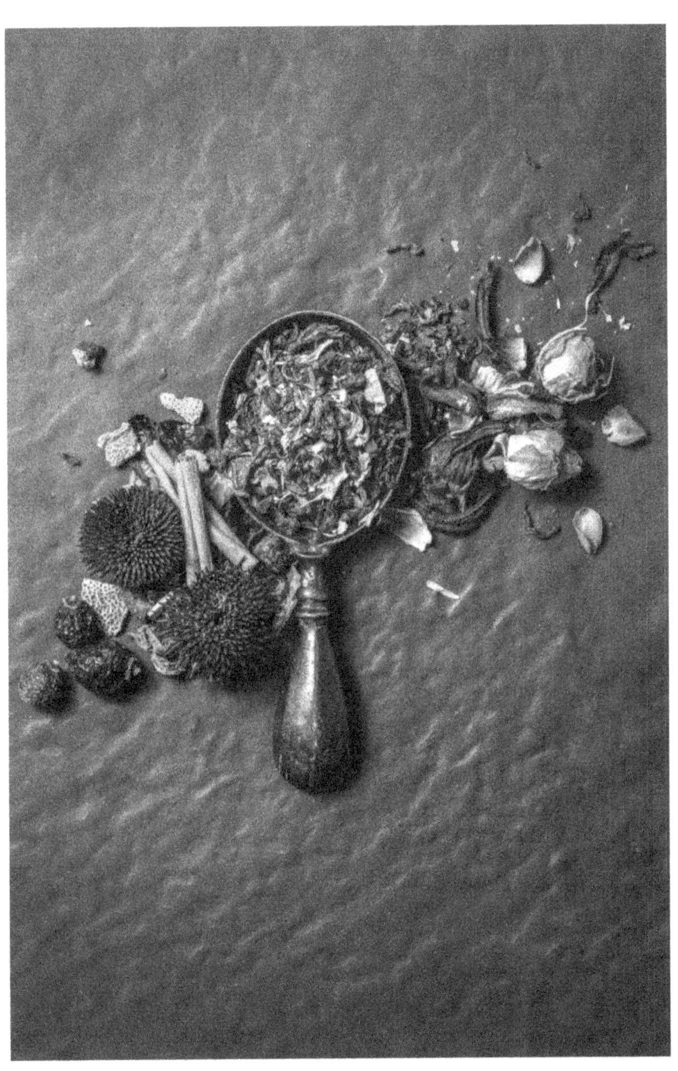

Conclusion

Natural Antibiotic and Antiviral Herbs' Future

Natural antibiotics and antiviral herbs have a promising future in terms of enhancing healthcare and battling infections. Here is a lengthy discussion of the field's future potential:

Ongoing scientific research is looking into the therapeutic potential of natural herbs as antibiotics and antivirals.

Researchers are researching the active molecules contained in herbs, how they work, and how they can aid with various ailments. This work gives a solid platform for future development and optimization of herbal medications.

Combination drugs: In the future, combination medicines that blend natural herbs with conventional antibiotics and antivirals may become available. Combining these approaches has the potential to improve overall therapeutic effectiveness and aid in the treatment of medication resistance. To deliver more effective and focused therapies, researchers are researching synergistic interactions between botanicals and conventional pharmaceuticals.

Standardization and Quality Control: The success of natural herbs as antibiotics and antivirals is contingent on improved standardization and quality control procedures.

Standardized processes for growing, harvesting, and processing herbs may help to assure consistency in potency and effectiveness. Quality control techniques, such as testing for pollutants and assuring purity, can improve the safety and dependability of herbal products even more.

Personalized treatment: With technology improvements and the study of individual genetic variations, personalized treatment is gaining prominence. In the future, healthcare experts may be able to personalize herbal medicines to an individual's exact genetic composition and health issues.

This tailored strategy can increase treatment outcomes while minimizing the probability of negative effects.

Alternative to Conventional Drugs: As worries about drug resistance and the negative effects of conventional antibiotics and antivirals develop, natural herbs may provide a viable alternative. Herbal medicines may be introduced into mainstream healthcare in the future, either as solo treatments or in conjunction with existing drugs. This integration can give a complete and personalized infection-control plan.

Health Promotion and Prevention: Natural herbs not only offer antibacterial effects, but they also promote overall health and well-being. Herbs for health promotion and prevention may receive more attention in the future.

Incorporating herbs into daily living, such as dietary habits and lifestyle choices, can contribute to the development of a strong immune system and minimize the risk of sickness.

Education and Awareness: The future of natural herbs as antibiotics and antivirals is contingent on boosting awareness and education among healthcare professionals and the general public.

Integrating herbal medicine material into medical and healthcare curricula supports practitioners in making educated decisions and recommendations. Furthermore, improving public understanding of the benefits, precautions, and proper use of herbal medicines encourages their safe and successful usage.

Sustainability and conservation: As the demand for natural herbs develops, it is necessary to address issues of sustainability and conservation.

To maintain the long-term availability of therapeutic herbs, the future will incorporate ethical cultivation, harvesting, and sourcing procedures. Sustainable cultivation methods, the protection of natural ecosystems, and the promotion of ethical sourcing practices will be crucial for the future of herbal medicine.

Ongoing research, customized treatment, combination medications, and greater education and awareness are all essential aspects that will have an impact on this sector. We can perhaps broaden treatment options, manage antibiotic resistance, and improve overall well-being by leveraging the potential of natural herbs and incorporating them into healthcare systems.

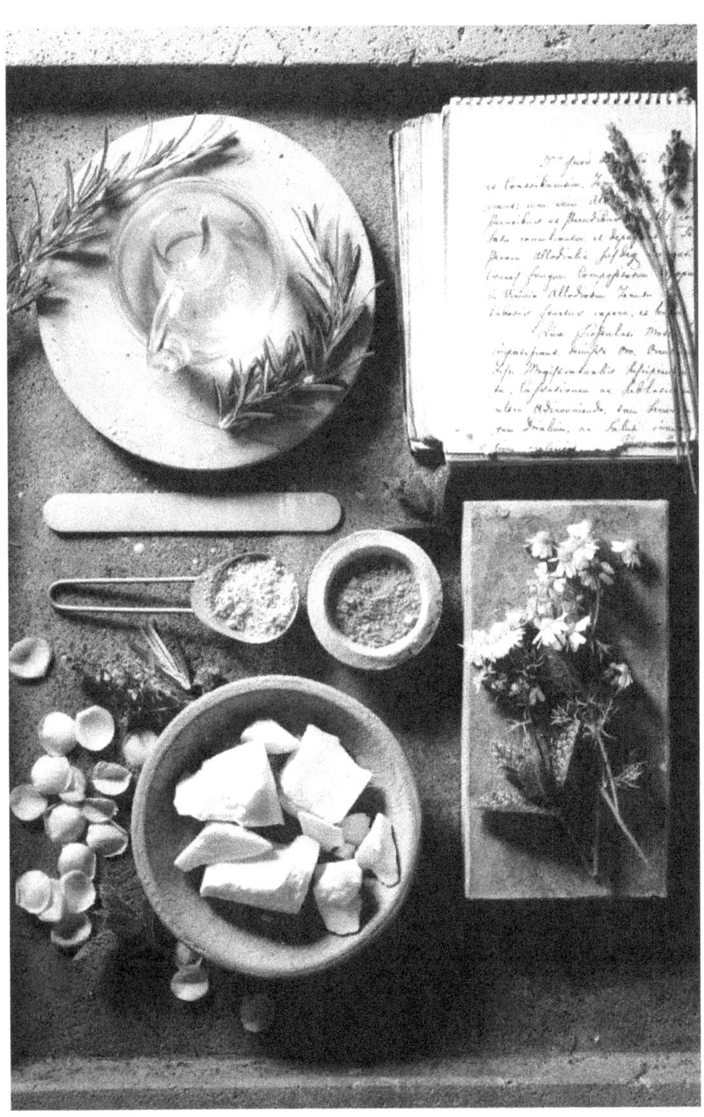